TABLE OF CONTENT

INTRODUCTION

Many traditional healers say that most of the healing is done by the patient and that every person has a responsibility for his or her proper behavior and health. This is a serious, lifelong responsibility. Healers serve as facilitators and counselors to help patients heal themselves. Healers use stories, humor, music, tobacco, smudging, and ceremonies to bring healing energies into the healing space and focus their effects. The healing process also goes beyond the individual patient. Traditional healers take into account not only the patient's immediate family and community, but future generations as well

Plants were carefully studied by the Native Americans over thousands of years contributing to the huge knowledge base of over 500 herbal plants. This plant and herbal knowledge learned and used by these early tribes was passed down orally for the most part as very little was written.

Many herbs that were discovered and used by Native Americans are used today and astonishingly used in the ways in which the Native Americans prescribed to using them.

MEDICINAL PLANTS THE NATIVE AMERICANS USED ON A DAILY BASIS

Native Americans are renowned for their medicinal plant knowledge. It is rumored they first started using plants and herbs for healing after watching animals eat certain plants when they were sick. In order to protect these plants from over harvesting, the medicine men used to pick every third plant they found.

The Native Americans had a spiritual view of life, and to be healthy, a person had to have a sense of purpose and follow a righteous, harmonious, and balanced path in life. They believed some illnesses were life lessons the person needed to learn and that they shouldn't interfere. Many modern remedies and medicines are based on the Native American knowledge of the different plants and herbs they used for thousands of years.

Here are the most versatile plants the Native Americans used in their everyday lives:

Yarrow (Achillea millefolium)

This fragrant, flowering plant has been used since Ancient Greece began using to stop excess bleeding. It is said the Greek hero Achilles used it on his wounds, hence the name. Pioneers and aboriginal people applied this on open wounds and cuts as a poultice made from the leaves to help clot the blood. They also combined fresh yarrow juice with water to help an upset stomach and for intestinal disorders. A tea made from the leaves and stems will act as an astringent.

Sumac

This plant can be used for multiple medicinal remedies, but it is one of the only plants that the healers used in treating eye problems. A decoction from sumac was used as a gargle to relieve sore throats or taken as a remedy for diarrhea. The leaves and berries were combined in tea to reduce fever or made into a poultice to soothe poison ivy.

Blackberry Ripe

The Cherokee used this plant for treating an upset stomach. They used blackberry tea for curing diarrhea and soothing swollen tissues and joints. An all-natural cough syrup to heal sore throats can be made from blackberry root mixed with honey or maple syrup. To soothe bleeding gums, they used to chew the leaves. This plant is also good for strengthening the whole immune system.

Rosemary

Native American tribes considered this plant sacred. They used it mostly as an analgesic for alleviating sore joints. This herb improves memory, relieves muscle pain and spasm, and helps the circulatory and the nervous systems. It also improves the immune system and treats indigestion.

Mint

The Cherokee used to make a mint tea to soothe digestion problems and help an upset stomach. They also made a salve from the leaves to relieve itching skin and rashes.

Red Clover

This plant has been used by healers for treating inflammation and respiratory conditions. Recent studies have shown that red clover helps to prevent heart disease by improving circulation and lowering cholesterol.

Black Gum

The Cherokee used to make a mild tea from the twigs and black gum bark to relieve chest pains.

Cattail

This is one of the most famous survival plants the indigenous population used for food but also as a preventative medicine. Because it's an easily digestible food, it's helpful for recovering from illness. It is called the supermarket of the swamp as it can be used in multiple dishes.

Pull Out a Sticker (Greenbriar)

This root tea was used as a blood purifier or for relieving joint pain. Some healers made a salve from leaves and bark mixed with hog lard, which was applied to minor sores, scalds, and burns.

Hummingbird Blossom (Buck Brush)

The Native Americans used this plant for treating mouth and throat conditions as well as cysts, fibroid tumors, and inflammation. It can be made into a poultice to help treat burns, sores, and wounds. A diuretic that stimulates kidney function can be made using the roots of this plant.

The early pioneers utilized this particular plant as a substitute for black tea. Recent studies have shown that hummingbird blossom is effective in treating high blood pressure and lymphatic blockages.

Wild Rose

The Native Americans used this plant as a preventive and a cure for a mild common cold. The tea stimulates the bladder and kidneys and is a mild diuretic. A petal infusion was used for a sore throat.

Saw Palmetto

The native tribes of Florida, such as the Seminoles, used the plant for food, but medicine men used it as a natural remedy for abdominal pain. It also helps digestion, reduces inflammation, and stimulates appetite.

Sage

Sage is commonly used as a spice, but it was a sacred plant for many indigenous tribes as it was thought to have effective purifying energies and to cleanse the body of negative energies. As a remedy, it was used for treating medical conditions like abdominal cramps, spasms, cuts, bruises, colds, and flu.

Wild Ginger

Healers used this plant for treating earache and ear infections. They also made a mild tea from the rootstock for stimulating the digestive system and relieving bloating. It also helps with bronchial infections and nausea.

Update: One of our readers sent us original pictures of wild ginger to help people identify the plant easier.

Slippery Elm

The Native Americans used the inner bark to fashion bow strings, rope, thread, and clothing. Tea was made from the bark and leaves to soothe toothaches, respiratory irritations, skin conditions, stomach ache, sore throats, and even spider bites.

Lavender

Healers used this plant as a remedy for insomnia, anxiety, depression, headache, and fatigue. The essential oil has antiseptic and anti-inflammatory properties. Infusions can be used to soothe insect bites as well as burns.

Prickly Pear Cactus

This is another plant that has been used as both a food and medicine. Native Americans made a poultice from mature pads as an antiseptic and for treating wounds, burns, and boils. Tea was made to treat urinary tract infections and to help the immune system. Now research shows that the prickly pear cactus helps to lower cholesterol and prevents diabetes and diet-related cardiovascular disease.

Honeysuckle

This plant has been used as a natural remedy by the Native Americans for treating asthma, but it has multiple healing purposes, including rheumatoid arthritis, mumps, and hepatitis. It also helps with upper respiratory tract infections, such as pneumonia.

Ashwagand -herb

This plant was an important plant for healers because of its many unusual medicinal uses. It treats bone weakness, muscle weakness and tension, loose teeth, memory loss, and rheumatism. It can also be used as a sedative. It has an overall rejuvenating effect on the body as it improves vitality. The leaves and the root bark can also be used as an antibiotic. If made into a poultice, it helps reduce swelling and treats pain. Caution is advised in the use of this plant since it is toxic.

Mullein

A tobacco-like plant, it was mainly used to treat respiratory disorders. The Native Americans made concoctions from the roots to reduce swelling in the joints, feet, or hands. Here you can find more medical uses for mullein.

Licorice Root

This root is famously used for flavoring candies, foods, and beverages. But it has also been used by healers to treat stomach problems, bronchitis, food poisoning, and chronic fatigue.

Uva Ursi

Because of the bear's affection toward this plant's fruits, it is also known as Bearberry and Beargrape. The Native Americans used this plant mainly for treating bladder and urinary tract infections.

Devil's Claw

Although the name would suggest a poisonous plant, the Native Americans used it to heal various conditions, from treating fever to soothing skin conditions, improving digestion, and treating arthritis. The tea can reduce the effects of diabetes, while a concoction made from the plant's roots reduces swelling and helps with joint disease, arthritis, gout, back pain, headache, and sores.

HEALING PLANTS

Native American, Alaska Native, and Native Hawaiian healers all have a long history of using indigenous, or native, plants for a wide variety of medicinal purposes. Medicinal plants and their applications are as diverse as the tribes who use them.

Beyond their medicinal benefits, indigenous plants were a staple of Native people's diet before Western contact. Today, indigenous plants are central to efforts to improve dietary health for current generations. In Hawai'i, the "Waianae Diet" and "Pre-Captain Cook Diet" aim to reduce empty calories, fat, and additives and promote a healthier, more balanced diet by restoring the role of indigenous foods. Alaska Natives and various Indian tribes have similar projects emphasizing traditional foods. In this very real sense, food is medicine.

Native Hawaiian Medicinal Plants

Hawaiian medicinal plants grow in many areas, including in the vicinity of heiaus or temples, sites that are considered sacred. In ancient times, Hawaiian traditional healers would practice La'au Lapa'au, medicinal healing, at some of the heiaus, using plants from around the heiau and in neighboring forests.

Most Hawaiian medicinal plants are foods that have additional curative properties. Healers view food as medicine, along with fresh, clean air and water. In all cases, healers offer a prayer to ask permission and give thanks for the medicines before harvesting and preparing them, and ask permission to facilitate medicinal healing on behalf of the Creator.

Hand-made, gray mortar and pestle.

Three-dimensional stone tool shaped into a circle with a flat bottom.

- Color image of a green aloe plant next to two large rocks.

- Color image of a green plant.

- Color image depicting the green leaves of a plantain plant.

- Color image depicting the green leaves of a banana plant. A thick, leafless stem is at the center of the image.

- Color image depicting the green leaves of a candlenut tree. Several candlenuts can be seen growing amongst the leaves.

- Color image of several palm trees standing tall in front of a blue sky, next to a few small houses.

- Color image of several green ginger plants growing in the wild. A few red-colored flowers can be seen growing amongst the green leaves of the plants.

- Color image of a guava plant. The light green guava fruit is growing in the middle of a few dark green leaves.

- Color image depicting several broad leaves of the Indian mulberry plant.

- Color image of several rocks of sea salt with an orange-brown hue.

- Color image of a green, leafy walhteria plant.

Southwest Indian Medicinal Plants

- Color photograph of a man in a white shirt and baseball cap standing in front of a few large yucca plants.

- Color image depicting the broad, spiky leaves of a mescal plant.

- Color image showing many thin, green leaves growing on the branches of a mesquite plant.

Upper Plains Indians Medicinal Plants

- Color image of a bee resting on the center of a purple coneflower.

- Color image of an uprooted bitterroot plant on a white background.

- Color image depicting several white and dark purple flowers of the osha plant.

Alaska Native Medicinal Plants

- Color image of a few devil's club leaves sprouting from the ground.

- Color image of a few, bright-yellow dandelion flowers surrounded by green grass.

- Color image depicting the branch of a willow tree, which is surrounded by several leafless plants.

11 POWERFUL NATIVE AMERICAN MEDICINAL CURES

The Cherokee is a Native American tribe that is indigenous to the Southeastern United States. They believe that the Creator has given them a gift of understanding and preserving medicinal herbs. The Cherokee trust the healing and preventative properties of nature's pharmacy. Because many plants become scarce throughout history, the Cherokee promote proper gathering techniques.

The old ones have taught them that if you are gathering, you should only pick every third plant you find. This ensures that enough specimens remain and will continue to propagate. Here are some of the medicinal plants that were commonly used and foraged for by the Cherokee tribe.

1. Blackberry

To the Cherokee, the blackberry is the longest known remedy to an upset stomach. However, this herb can be used for just about anything. Using a strong tea from the root of blackberry helps to reduce swelling of tissue and joints. A decoction of the roots, sweetened with honey or maple syrup, makes an excellent cough syrup. Even chewing on the leaves of blackberry can soothe bleeding gums. (source)

Some other health benefits of blackberry fruit include

- better digestion

- strengthened immune system

- healthy functioning of the heart

- prevention of cancer

- relief from endothelial dysfunction

These tasty berries are also incredibly nutritious. Vitamins provided by blackberries include vitamin A, vitamin B6, vitamin C, vitamin E, vitamin K, thiamine, riboflavin, niacin, and folate. Blackberries also have an incredible mineral wealth of calcium, iron, magnesium, phosphorous, potassium, and zinc. They are also an excellent source of dietary fiber and essential amino acids.

2. Hummingbird Blossom (Buck Brush)

The Cherokee has used hummingbird blossom for the treatment of cysts, fibroid tumors, inflammation, and mouth/throat problems. Present day research has concluded that this herb is also ideal for treating high blood pressure and lymphatic blockages. (source)

The Cherokee mainly use hummingbird blossom as a diuretic to stimulate kidney function; however, it was also used to treat conditions such as:

- Inflamed tonsils

- Enlarged lymph nodes

- Enlarged spleens

- Hemorrhoids

- Menstrual bleeding.

To get all of the benefits from hummingbird blossom, the Cherokee would steep the leave and flowers in boiling water for about five minutes then drink the tea while it is still warm.

3. Cattail

The Cherokee consider this herb to not exactly be a healing medicine, but rather a preventative medicine. It is an easily digestible food that can help with recovery from illnesses. Almost every part of this herb, except for the mature leaves and seed heads, can be used for medicinal purposes. The root of cattail is high in starch, and the male plants are high in pollen content.

Cattail root can be prepared much like potatoes, boiled and mashed. The resulting paste is a great remedy for burns and sores. The pollen from cattail is a great source of protein and can be used as a supplement in baking. The fuzz from flowers called the seed down can also be used to prevent skin irritation in babies, such as diaper rash. The flowers of cattail can even be eaten to help with diarrhea.

4. Pull Out a Sticker (Greenbriar)

The roots of this herb are high in starch while the leaves and stems are rich in various vitamins and minerals. Due to the rubbery texture of Greenbriar, its roots can be used like potatoes. The starch in the root of Greenbriar has a harsh, strange taste but is rich in calories.

The Cherokee use Greenbriar as a blood purifier and mild diuretic that treats urinary infections. Many Cherokee healers make an ointment from the leaves and bark and apply it to minor sores and burns. The leaves from this herb can even be used in your tea to treat arthritis! The berries of Greenbrier can be eaten raw or made into jams. They make great vegan jello shots too.

5. Mint

Mint is a very popular herb in present day culture and is commonly used in tea. However, many people don't know that mint contains a variety of antioxidant properties. It also contains magnesium, phosphorus potassium, calcium, vitamin C, vitamin A, and fiber!

The Cherokee use this herb to aid with digestion. (1) The leaves can be crushed and used as cold compresses, made into ointments, and even added to your bath to sooth itchy skin. The Cherokee healers use a blend of stems and leaves to lower high blood pressure. If you are breastfeeding and find your nipples cracking, try applying some mint water. It worked miracles for me!

6. Mullein

This herb has the power to soothe asthma and chest congestion. According to the Cherokee, inhaling the smoke from burning mullein roots and leaves works miracles to calm your lungs and open up pathways. Mullein is exceptionally helpful to soothe the mucous membranes.

You can make a warm decoction and soak your feet in it to reduce swelling and joint pain. Due to mullein's anti-inflammatory properties, it soothes painful and irritated tissue. Mullein flowers can be used to make tea which has mild sedative effects.

7. Qua lo ga (Sumac)

Every single part of this herb can be utilized for medicinal purposes! Sumac bark can be made into a mild decoction that can be taken to soothe diarrhea. The decoction of the bark can also be gargled to help with a sore throat. Ripe berries can make a pleasant beverage that is rich in Vitamin C.

The tea from the leaves of sumac can reduce fevers. You can even crush the leaves into an ointment to help relieve a poison ivy rash. A study published in Iranian Journal of Pharmaceutical Research reported that sumac if added to the daily diet, can help lower cholesterol levels (source).

8. Big Stretch (Wild Ginger)

The Cherokee recommend a mild tea, made from the root of wild ginger, to stimulate better digestion. This herb can also help with intestinal gas, upset stomach, and colic. A strong tea from the root of wild ginger can be used to remove secretion from the lungs.

The Meskwaki, another Native American tribe, use crushed, steeped stems of wild ginger as a relief from earaches. You can use rootstocks from this herb as a substitute for regular ginger and flowers as the flavoring for your favorite recipe!

9. Jisdu Unigisdi (Wild Rose)

The fruit of a wild rose is a rich source of vitamin C and is a great remedy for the common cold and the flu. The Cherokee would make a mild tea out of wild rose hips to stimulate bladder and kidney function. You can even make your own petal infusion to soothe a sore throat! Or try making a decoction from the root to help with diarrhea. My grandmother uses to make jam out of the petals and it was delicious.

10. Squirrel Tail (Yarrow)

This herb is known best for its blood clotting properties. Fresh, crushed leaves can be applied to open wounds to stop excess bleeding. Yarrow's juice, mixed with spring water, can stop internal bleeding from stomach and intestinal illnesses. You can also use the leaves to make tea which will stimulate abdominal functions and assist in proper digestion.

It can also help with kidney and gallbladder related issues. Oh, and did I mention that you can use a decoction made from leaves and stems to help improve your acne? It works wonders for chapped hands and other skin irritations.

11. Kawi Iyusdi (Yellow Dock)

The Cherokee often use this herb in their kitchen. It is very similar to spinach but contains a lot more vitamins and minerals due to its long roots that gather nutrients from deep underground. The leaves of yellow dock are a great source of iron and can also be used as a laxative. (

You can even prepare a juice decoction out of yellow dock stems from treating minor sores, diaper rash, and itching. The Cherokee healers use a decoction, made from the crushed roots of yellow dock, as a warm wash for its antiseptic properties.

You should always remember that all of the above-mentioned medicinal plants are very potent and might be dangerous if used in the wrong way. The Cherokee healers have many centuries of practice and experience. Another thing to keep in mind is the fact that these herbs are all very valuable! They are the nature's pharmacy, so please be kind and caring when scavenging any of these.

This information is not intended to be a substitute for professional medical advice, diagnosis or treatment. Always seek the advice of your physician or other ⬚ualified health provider with any questions about your medical condition and/or current medication. Do not disregard professional medical advice or delay seeking advice or treatment because of something you have read here.

THE MIND-BODY HEALING LINK

HOW TO RESTORE AND REPAIR

According to conventional wisdom, confronting illness is nothing short of an act of war: We battle cancer or fight colds, shielding the body from nasty foreign invaders, usually in the form of pathogens (read: germs) that threaten to colonize us with disease.

In response, we send out troops in the form of antibodies (including a regiment actually called "natural killer cells") to defend our native territory.

If the good guys win, our health prevails. If the bad guys win, we're sick.

But the newest way to think about healing (which also, coincidentally, is the oldest way) is how to nurture what's good rather than destroying what's bad a matter of plowshares, not swords.

Servan-Schreiber, a neuroscientist, helped usher in the use of cutting-edge technology to catch images of the brain in the act of thinking, and his expertise around cancer and healing comes from personal as well as clinical experience.

A Surprising Discovery

Eighteen years ago, when a volunteer subject turned out to be a no-show, Servan-Schreiber stepped into an MRI scanner himself -- and discovered his own brain tumor.

Surgery and chemotherapy helped him into remission, but when he asked his oncologist what he could do to help prevent a relapse, his doctor had no answer. So he dedicated himself to learning how diet and lifestyle changes could boost his inner healing resources. (His cancer remains in remission today.)

"We all have natural mechanisms for ongoing healing in our bodies," he explains, and conducting our everyday lives in ways that nurture those mechanisms is a key part of preventing and recovering from illness.

Not to say that conventional medicine doesn't have its place -- especially when it comes to cancer. "You cannot replace chemotherapy with broccoli, jogging, and meditation," he says, "but it's clear that those three things change the way your genes control biology."

The Biology of Healing

Even healing from a cut isn't just a matter of isolated tissues knitting back together. As soon as you nick your hand, several systems launch into action: The clotting system of the blood immediately forms a fibrin clot to stop the bleeding. The circulatory and cardiovascular systems start delivering white blood cells to fend off bacteria and protect the wound from infection while also delivering cells called fibroblasts, which lay down collagen to aid in tissue repair.

And the stress response kicks in, controlling the normal operations of the body -- such as inflammation, digestion, and elimination -- to divert resources (like blood flow) toward the crisis.

So not only is healing happening all the time, it's also happening all over the body, which is why you can do more to aid the healing of a cut than slap on a bandage.

Research shows, for example, that good nutrition speeds wound healing and that moderate exercise can aid in circulation (which brings in oxygen and nutrients and washes out toxins).

She'd spent her career studying the seminal links between stress in the brain, inflammation, and rheumatoid arthritis. And then she developed inflammatory arthritis, a similar condition, herself.

Sternberg blames a taxing combination of stress from long hours in the lab and grief over her mother's death for triggering her own illness. It was only when she accepted an invitation to spend some time at a friend's home in Greece that she learned firsthand the effects of destressing on mind and body.

After just a few days of long walks through the countryside, delicious, fresh Mediterranean food, and plenty of rest, she noticed improvements in her condition that surprised her.

"I was watching some fishermen down on their boats one afternoon, and I felt how connected they were to the rhythms of the sun and the sea," she recalls. "That was the moment when I realized I'd been doing it all wrong. I needed to change my way of living if I was going to continue to get better."

This profound personal experience not only informed her own health, but changed the way she viewed healing. "Every moment of the day, we deal with insults to our emotional, physical, and spiritual selves," she explains.

Those insults can come in the form of cuts and scrapes, viruses, allergens, junk food, muscle strains, anxiety, heartbreak, and more.

The Mind-Body Link

Once considered a radical idea in Western medicine, the mind's power over the body has garnered considerable respect over the past couple of decades, thanks to a growing body of neurological research and new technologies, such as functional MRIs.

Researchers have established that biochemical, released from the brain during various mood states, affect how well the body repairs itself.

Negative feelings (such as anxiety, fear, and loneliness) have been shown to trigger stress hormones such as cortisol and epinephrine, which inhibit the immune system, while positive feelings (like happiness, love, and peacefulness) can boost our healing ability through feel-good neurotransmitters such as dopamine and oxytocin.

The research shows that this isn't all light and fairy dust, either: A study from Pittsburgh's Carnegie Mellon University suggests that positive emotions may aid in warding off the common cold. When 334 ▢uarantined volunteers were infected with a cold virus, those who tended to experience positive emotions (feeling content and relaxed) were more likely to resist infection and avoid developing symptoms than those who tended toward depression, hostility, and anxiety.

Research shows that depression, which affects cortisol levels, can worsen outcomes in patients with cancer and heart disease, while loneliness and social isolation have been linked to weakened immune systems, high blood pressure, and faster progression of Alzheimer's disease.

Explaining the Placebo Effect

There's perhaps no better proof of the impact of mind over matter than the placebo effect. Studies suggest that it accounts for around 30 percent of the response to any medical intervention and yet has been traditionally dismissed by researchers as some kind of magical thinking. In fact, it's a powerful example of the connection between thoughts, beliefs, and physical healing.

"The placebo effect is not a sham," Sternberg says. "It's evidence that the brain plays a very important role in healing." When we expect a pill or treatment to help us, Sternberg explains, the brain shifts gears, "releasing endorphins and other chemicals that support the immune system in its job."

The great news about healing is that our minds and bodies know intrinsically how to do it -- if only we'd allow them.

"Unfortunately, in the past 60 years or so, we've developed a number of habits that get in the way of our natural healing mechanism," Servan-Schreiber says. Our diet, for instance, has shifted away from whole foods and toward processed nutrient-deficient, low-fiber, high-sugar foods that trigger cellular inflammation, which, he says, "makes it hard for our body's natural defenses to take hold" -- and easier for cancer and other diseases to gain control. Reduced immune function is also associated with a sedentary lifestyle and increased isolation and depression.

"It's not a single stressor that makes you sick," Sternberg says. It's the cumulative effect of many stressors on the body, mind, and spirit that wear you down and make you vulnerable. We consulted a range of experts for their healing strategies and have come up with six key lifestyle changes to keep your self-healing systems vital -- and intact.

6Ways to Boost Healing

1. Ease Stress with Pleasure

When people tell Sternberg that they don't have time to get a massage or sit in the park for lunch, she asks, "Do you have time to be sick?" Relaxation and pleasure are healing states of mind, she says, and if we don't visit them regularly, we compromise the body's ability to recover from its daily traumas.

Anything you can do to reduce your stress response will pay off on the healing front: A 2010 study on post-traumatic stress disorder (PTSD), headed by Columbia University's Mailman School of Public Health, suggests that severe stress can alter one's genetics and affect the body's immune function for years to come. PTSD has long been associated with compromised physical health, including diabetes and heart disease.

Seek out stimulation. Admiring a work of art, listening to music, or tending a garden aren't just extracurricular but part of a comprehensive health-insurance plan. Sternberg says doing things you enjoy triggers the brain to release feel-good chemicals.

Make love. Not only is sex a fine idea in general, it also replenishes stress-relieving hormones and, according to researchers at Wilkes University in Pennsylvania, beefs up the immune system by increasing levels of the antibody IgA, which protects against colds and other infections. Of 111 subjects, those who reported having sex once or twice a week had higher levels of IgA in their saliva than those who abstained, had sex less than once a week, or had it three times or more. (So there can be too much of a good thing!)

2. Find Something to Believe In

Research indicates that people who have a spiritual faith of some kind are better equipped to deal with illness. A recent study from the University of Miami shows that patients with HIV who described themselves as "spiritual" (meaning they have a sense of peace, faith in God, or a compassionate view of others) showed a higher count of AIDS-fighting CD4 immunity cells and a lower viral load.

3. Talk It Out

It's true: Hostility is bad for your health. Studies show it can raise levels of cytokines, behavior-regulating proteins in the immune system that are associated with arthritis, osteoporosis, and other conditions.

A 2005 study from Ohio State University looked at the effect of marital discord on simple wound healing in 42 married couples. Researchers found that couples who "demonstrated consistently higher levels of hostile behaviors" healed 40 percent more slowly from their lab-inflicted blister wounds than the more harmonious couples. When the subjects attended a structured interaction to help moderate conflict, their wound healing improved.

Don't bite your tongue. A 10-year study published in Psychosomatic Medicine found that wives who silenced themselves during arguments with their husbands were four times more likely to die during that period than women who spoke their minds; they were also more likely to suffer from depression and irritable bowel syndrome. Learning conflict resolution skills can help self-silencers to speak up. If you aren't ready to express your problems aloud, get those emotions out some other way: Write them down or even have a private venting session.

4. Get to Bed

"Sleep and immune health are inextricably linked" Many of the body's major restorative functions --tissue repair, muscle growth, protein synthesis -- happen mostly or exclusively during sleep, and studies have linked sleep deprivation with lowered immune ability and increased obesity and inflammation, all of which are risk factors for heart disease, cancer, and stroke. Everyone's sleep needs vary, but most adults re□uire between seven and nine hours per night.

Change your attitude about sleep. "People who sleep well love sleep. The key then, he says, is falling in love with it. Create a few pleasurable bedtime rituals (take a hot bath with lavender oil, turn off electronics). Skip the nightly glass of Pinot, though, as alcohol before bed tends to increase wakefulness during the night.

A regular daily yoga practice may also reduce stress and encourage better sleep. One new study shows that cancer survivors who practiced gentle yoga twice a week reported a 22 percent improvement in sleep quality and cut their use of sleep medication by an average of 21 percent.

5. Eat Plenty of Healing Foods

Create an inner healing environment by feeding your body nutrients that boost immune function and lower inflammation. Nutritionist and naturopathic doctor Cathy Wong, author of "The Inside-Out Diet," offers her favorites:

Get your fruits and veggies. No surprise here: A range of colorful fruits and vegetables provides you with vitamins and minerals, plus disease- fighting antioxidants. Try apples, oranges, tomatoes, berries, and dark-green vegetables (broccoli, kale, collard greens).

Enhance your immunity. Protein provides the amino acids that are the building blocks of the immune system; lean meat also contains iron, zinc, and vitamins B6 and B12. Try wild salmon and lean turkey and chicken; vegetarian options include beans and legumes (lentils, chickpeas, kidney beans), nuts, and seeds (try sunflower and pumpkin).

Turn down the sugar dial. Opt for foods low in sugar to help reduce inflammation, such as artichokes, oatmeal, brown rice, and beans, which have a high ratio of fiber to sugar. Try a natural sweetener such as stevia, which has a more muted effect on blood-glucose levels than cane sugar or even honey.

Get enough good bugs. he gastrointestinal tract plays a critical role in the immune response because its large surface area comes into contact with so many microorganisms and potential pathogens. Eating fermented foods promotes beneficial bacteria, or probiotics, in the digestive system, crowding out disease-causing bacteria and keeping them out of the bloodstream. Add fermented foods to your diet by eating yogurt, kefir, miso, tempeh, and even (unpasteurized) pickles and sauerkraut.

6. Move It

It's hard to overstate the benefits of being physically fit: Regular moderate exercise promotes circulation, strengthens heart muscles, and increases nutrient delivery and oxygenation of cells -- all of which are critical for healthy immune function. New genetic studies also suggest that exercise helps keep cells healthy by protecting the telomeres, or tips of DNA, that are involved with gene replication. But there's another healing aspect of exercise that Eastern cultures recognize. "In Chinese medicine, exercise is considered an activation of chi, or energy flow, which can, in turn, improve one's ability to fight disease and heal," Ni says.

Keep it short and sweet. For the best results and the least wear and tear on muscles and joints, try working out in frequent, shorter sessions (say, 30 minutes of walking, dancing, yoga, or other mild aerobic exercise three to four times a week) rather than marathon workouts once or twice a week. In terms of immunity, it's just as important not to overdo it: "You'll know you've over exercised if you're exhausted after each workout, get frequent colds and flus, or are always in pain due to your effort,

HOW GARDENS HEAL YOUR BODY, MIND, AND SPIRIT

Amidst my whirlwind workday, a sniff of an herb in the garden outside my store reminded me of my grandmother, from South Africa, who passed recently. She is the one who started me on the path of becoming a professional urban farmer, gardener, educator, and entrepreneur, and random moments like this strike often. I stood still and allowed the fragrance to envelop me, and to bask in her memory. In that moment of reflection, calm washed over me, and I knew that, once again, the garden was serving to heal.

The definition of healing is broad and touches many parts of our lives. According to the Merriam-Webster dictionary, healing means:

1a: to make sound or whole, b: to restore to health;

2a: to cause (an undesirable condition) to be overcome, b: to patch up (a breach or division);

3: to restore to original purity or integrity. Gardens heal in many surprising ways, and it is exciting to see the positive healing effects they are having in places as diverse as corporate head□uarters, children's hospitals, senior centers, and city halls. Healing effects can be seen in many ways, including these:

1. Gardens can serve as a place for reflection for those needing comfort. People carry their personal worries with them all day long concerns about their ailing parent, struggling child, financial challenges, or fears about the future. Peaceful moments in gardens, where the sensual joys of plants growing can inspire feelings of hope, serve to counteract those stresses. What's more, when faced with acute stress resulting from the recent death of a loved one or a significant tragedy covered 24/7 by the news media; there is something very life-affirming about planting a seed and seeing it grow. In fact, it has been said that planting a seed is the ultimate act of faith in the future.

2. Gardens can provide plants that have actual medicinal uses. It's sometimes easy to forget that our modern medicine originated in plant-based medicinal therapies. The continual surge of interest in herbal medicine and home remedies is a reminder of the abundant healing benefits of our natural world. Simple herbal possibilities such as a cup of peppermint tea to energize, some lemon balm to aid digestion, or the sniff of a sprig of lavender to encourage sleep can easily become a welcome healthy habit in everyday life for those with a small herb garden. More extensive medicinal uses of a wide variety of plants can be learned as well. (Note: Do not consider this medical advice, and tell your doctor if you are using any herbs in addition to prescribed medication.)

3. Gardens can enable those on the edges of society to feel connected. In this context, healing may mean assuaging feelings of disconnect from society, and gardens have been shown to be valuable tools in helping everyone from seniors to incarcerated youth feel not only useful but necessary. Gardens can showcase hidden skills and teach new ones, provide responsibility that gives individuals a reason to keep showing up, and forge healthy relationships and connections across generations in non-threatening environments.

4. Gardens can help restore the earth. Let's not overlook the fact that organically-grown gardens don't only hold the potential of healing people but also our planet. They sequester carbon, mitigate water runoff, filter environmental toxins, increase biological diversity, encourage ecosystem development, and enhance the beauty, vitality, and even safety of our communities. Many municipalities are getting into the garden action because of these almost immediately seen results in which adding a little extra green space grows the health and welfare of their cities, counties, and states.

As you consider the value of your garden, don't overlook the simple and significant healing benefits that it affords you. If you would be so kind, please share with us how you have found gardens to be healing as your words may be exactly what someone else needs to hear right now.

HEALING MIND POWER

HOW IT WORKS

I've heard the same conversations over and over. Just sitting on the train every morning, passengers on the phone, or chatting with friends unencumbered by those around them, talking about their problems. The girl whose boyfriend left and is now perpetually lethargic and depressed; the woman whose mother or grandmother died of breast cancer and wakes up every day in fear of the disease; and let's not forget the man who stands confidently in a carriage full of passengers who are sneezing and coughing with winter flu, while he resolutely states 'I never get sick' and he never ever appears to. Ah, I know these people well and if there is one thing I could tell them it would be this- The mind is a powerful thing. Healing mind power is not a myth, but a distinct possibility.

How is the mind connected to the brain, what is its purpose and how does it effect the body? Philosophers and scientists have spent decades trying to understand the complex mind-body connection under the banner of psychoneuroimmunology, psychophysiology, neuropsychology. One thing is certain; the mind is far more powerful than we often give it credit. Deepak Chopra recently tweeted of a neuroscientist who once said "The brain is so complicated it staggers its own imagination." We have often heard stories of a woman lifting a car to rescue her child underneath, or a paralyzed man willing himself to walk again. These cases and many more have been termed as medical miracles because such is the power of the mind that it can stimulate adrenaline at will and heal damaged tissue in the body.

To understand how to heal with the mind you must first understand how the mind affects the body. Science shows that the nervous system in the body acts as a communication pathway between every cell and organ. Like a perfect WiFi connection, neurotransmitters send signals everywhere in response to our thoughts and feelings. This interaction is probably better understood when you or I become stressed. On the first day of a job, or proposing to a girl- the hands become sweaty, the blood pressure rises and the heart races along like a V12. Waves of emotion have a phenomenal effect on our body at these crucial times, but what's happening to us when the current is calmer? What are we telling our bodies with every slow and constant lap of the water against the shore?

Every tidal wave begins with just one small ripple somewhere in the ocean, and it is not surprising that a large number of medical studies demonstrate that negative emotions play a significant role in the development of heart disease, chronic pain and cancer. So if our thoughts can cause us illness, surely they can get us out of the same mess. Positive thing and optimistic beliefs have been shown to enhance healing processes. Similarly the placebo effect is widely used in medicine to produce a beneficial improvement in a patients' health who believes that they are being treated with a real medical drug rather than an inactive substance. The patients' expectation to improve is so strong that it can affect the body and there-in lies the secret and key to health and happiness.

Consistent thought processes, such as fear, forgiveness, hate and anger can manifest as physical ailments but these can also be changed and the body healed by creating new thought patterns by the use of affirmations. It is important to first find the root of the problem and that means turning off the numerous distractions the world has to offer and tuning within- to those feelings you push to the back of your mind, to those fears you are afraid to speak of but lace the words of your everyday conversations.

SECRETS OF MIND POWER TO ULTIMATE HEALTH

Being in a state of excellent health is more than eating healthily and exercising regularly. We all know that we can get sick if we are stressed or tired but the connection between the mind and the body and the ability of the mind to heal the body and keep it healthy is a lot more profound than many people think.

The mind essentially is the body and the opposite applies too. There is nowhere in the body that the mind does not exist and it is only in recent years that scientists are starting to recognize this connection albeit on a limited level at present. But what you may ask does this mean for us and how can we use the mind to experience better health in our lives?

One of the obvious areas that people have trouble with when it comes to their health is the area in maintaining a healthy weight and mind power can play a very active role here if you use it wisely. One of the most profound things that you can do is to simply use your mind to become more aware of when you are full and have had enough to eat.

Many of us eat unconsciously and consume too much food but if you focus your attention on how full you feel you will find yourself eating less and losing weight.

We can also focus our mind on how we are feeling at the time when we are hungry. Many of us eat emotionally i.e. when we feel bored or sad, and not because we are truly hungry, and you can learn when you actually need the need emotional substance rather than food sustenance by simply using the mind and paying attention.

Most of the ailments that we experience in our lives can also be eased and healed with the proper use of our mind. The body is in essence a physical representation of the mind and when we get ill it can simply be the body's way of telling us that we are not paying attention to something that is going on in our mind.

One way to start the healing process using our mind power is to focus on paying attention and locating which part of our body which is having trouble. Then start talking to that specific body part and have an internal dialogue with it.

Because the body is inextricably linked with the mind, it can react positively to these dialogues.

Another main health problem that's common is when we are feeling stressed, be it in our work, life or relationship, we tend to fall sick easily. If we want to achieve optimal health, then we should work on cultivating peace and harmony in our minds. One of the best ways to achieve this is through meditation, where you learn how to still the mind and calm it. When we focus our mind power on learning how to still and quieten the mind with exercises such as these we can really start to take control of our lives and experience ultimate health gains as well.

NATURAL HEALING FOR THE BODY

Back-to-Nature Aromatherapy

Back-to-nature is a new health initiative by people living in modern society. Aromatherapy, which stems from natural plants, has also became a favorite in modern day living. Ancient medical healers use essential oils to heal people's bodies and aroma to soothe their spirits. As whiffs of fragrance drift through the ages of time, people living in modern society have even made use of the latest scientific research to develop the unlimited potential and precious deposits of essential oils, so as to improve the environment, enhance healthiness and beautify the spirit.

Aromatherapy comes from the essence of natural flora and enters the human body though the air and the olfactory nerves. From there, it goes though the central nerves into our brains and, tapping on the characteristics of plants hormones, it is able to deliver beneficial effects to the body, such as the lungs, blood, emotional nerves, immune system and even aid in psychological aspects such as the alleviation or pacification of problems like depression.

Aromatherapy uses a simple natural method to kill bacteria and increase nutrients in the air that we breathe. At the same time, aromatherapy is able to allow the surrounding environment to create anions which are extremely good for the human body. Different plant fragrances will create different feelings and responses in our body. Aromatherapy uses the characteristics of plant essential oils to improve the health and balance between complexion, body, cognition and spirit, so as to achieve a state where the body, heart and spirit become one.

The Genie of Aroma - Plant Essential Oils

All plants will go through photosynthesis where the cells will secrete aromatic molecules. These molecules will assemble into aromatic pouches dispersed on the petals, leaves or branches. After extracting these aromatic pouches, we will get what we term as plant essential oils.

The essential oils used by aromatherapy can be said to be the hormones of plants. They have the same building components and life energy as human beings. Essential oils are made from the amalgamation of different kind of molecules. These molecules exist together, in a beautiful proportion. As molecules are very fine and have high penetration ability, they can effectively enter the body and not leave behind any toxins.

According to research, pure plant essential oils will not be like chemical pharmaceuticals that remain in the body. They will utilize the body's excretory system such as urine, perspiration and breathing to purge out of the body. If the usage is correct, natural essential oils will have no side effects.

The natural aroma of plant essential oils, after entering into the brain via the olfactory nerves, is able to stimulate the frontal brain to secrete some hormones, so as to give a most comfortable state of mind. This is the best way to protect the spirit. One is also able to group different essential oils together to blend an aroma to one's liking. This will not damage the characteristics of essential oils and will even empower their functions.

The basic characteristics of essential oils can prevent contagious diseases and fight bacteria, pathogens and moulds. They can also prevent inflammation and convulsion as well as enhance cellular metabolism and regenerating abilities, making life even better. These essential oils can also regulate the inner secretion organs, enhancing the secretion of hormones and enabling the physiological and psychological activities of the body to develop well. Essential oils can even relax the nerves, enhance blood circulation, reduce depression, make one happier and enable cognition and psychology to reach a harmonious state.

The Functions of Phytoncidere:

1. Eliminates bacteria.

2. Purifies air of pollutants to ensure smoother breathing for greater vitality.

3. Enters the body via the nasal passage to fight diseases and maintain physical and mental balance.

Scientific Research of Aromatherapy

Aromatherapy is a method that premises on the absorption of active materials to heal, alleviate and prevent various diseases and contagion. It can activate vigorous elements in the body to fight all pathogen elements, achieving the effect of healing and boosting of the immune system.

Aroma psychology that arises out of "Aroma Healing Studies" is a science that specifically examines the psychological state and inner responses that occur when one inhales perfume. It uses experiments and the results of various measuring instruments to prove the effects of aromatherapy. It is able to present the research results in a quantitative manner and enable aromatherapy to go the way of science.

Effects of Anion:

1. Respiratory system: anions can enhance the fine hair activities in the nose sticky membrane, windpipe and bronchus sticky membrane; elevate the expansion of smooth muscles; help in the elimination of phlegmatic liquids; soothe the sensitive reactions of the respiratory system and is especially helpful to nose sensitivity.

2. Blood circulation system: lowers blood pressure, slows the heart rate, reduces the precipitation speed of red blood cells, lengthens the time for blood to coagulate and aids in the smooth circulation of blood.

3. Immune System: activates the dermis system function, elevates protein contents in the blood cells, hence increasing the ability to fight diseases.

4. Control bacteria in the air and reduce diseases to do with the respiratory organs.

5. Adjust and regulate the active response functions of the nervous system, hence soothing feelings of anxiety and uneasiness.

How Essential Oils Are Absorbed by the Human Body

Essential oils are absorbed by the body through two channels, the skin and the lungs. The skin is originally endowed with the functions of absorption and excretion. Essential oils molecules are very tiny and are able to penetrate into the skin and in between the lymph and cells, and then spread to the blood in other parts of the body. Absorption method happens via the pulmonary alveoli in the lungs, into the surrounding capillary bloodstream and is able to release refined plant hormones into the air through aromatherapy, allowing the body to absorb quickly and achieve therapeutic benefits.

When the lungs absorb phytoncidere nutrients, it is not only healthy for the lungs; it will also forge a healthy connection between the lungs and the heart, as well as the heart and the blood vessels. So, after the lungs absorb this large amount of nutrients, it will send these nutrients to the heart, and the heart will then send these nutrients to the blood vessels, which will then send the nutrients to every cell in the human body!

10 WAYS TO RESTORE ENERGY

You have the power to cultivate energy within your body in any moment. Even when you're exhausted, burned out and feel like you've got nothing left to give, your body can guide you to a space of greater vitality, inner strength and wellbeing.

Here are some strategies that I've used in my own life to do just that:

1. Rest when your body says rest.

It's important to follow your body's cues on when you need to rest rather than pushing yourself beyond what you can handle and then crashing. If in doubt, rest. When you listen to your body and give yourself the rest you need, you'll rebuild your energy over the long-term.

2. Cultivate stillness within you.

There's an incredible healing power in stillness. Prioritize creating quiet spaces in your day where you can simply be still. Really allow yourself to feel the stillness around you, letting it soak into your body. Notice that you too, that you also hold a stillness within the core of who you are.

3. Practice whole-body breathing.

Each day, take time out to breathe consciously. Feel your breath inside your body and notice how far it reaches within you. With each inhalation and exhalation, feel your breath extend further into your body (until it feels like every cell in your whole body is breathing). Then relish that feeling of life within your body.

4. Nourish your body wholeheartedly.

Be conscious and heartfelt in how you nourish your body by choosing foods that feel inherently good for you. Notice which foods provide a sense of restoration and healing in your body. And if you're unsure, ask your innermost self what your body needs in this moment.

5. Explore gentle and restorative movement.

Integrating gentle movement into your day can help you connect more fully with your body and self. Light walking, stretching, restorative yoga, and similar activities can be wholly supportive of you regaining energy in your body and life. Explore various types of movement and see what feels right for your body.

6. Have compassion for your self.

We gain energy from love and compassion. Be gentle with yourself when you're exhausted, and treat yourself kindly. Be kind in your thoughts and feelings towards your self as well as in your actions. Feel love and compassion in your heart and extend that warmth to yourself regularly.

7. Stop doing what drains you.

You'll instantly feel lighter and more alive when you choose to stop doing what drains you. Be aware of how your body responds to various things, people, places and experiences in your life; genuinely consider whether they support and fulfill you, or deplete you of energy.

8. Nurture what inspires you.

The feeling of inspiration is energizing in itself. Get clear on what truly inspires you by checking for that feeling of energy deep in your body. It may show up as a burning desire or an inner knowledge of your truth, but once you've found it, feed and nurture it through your thoughts, energy, and actions.

9. Be vigilant with your time.

Learn to guard your time like the precious gift that it is. Choose wisely in how you spend it, ensuring that you schedule plenty time and space to care for yourself. Don't be quick to give it away, but when you do, be sure to give it willingly from a place of wholeheartedness.

10. Look for a deeper meaning.

When you can see meaning in your experience of exhaustion or burnout, you'll instantly feel lighter. Get curious about the lesson in this challenging time. When you do, you'll feel a genuine appreciation for your experiences, knowing that you'll grow and evolve as a result, and be able to contribute more fully to this world.

25 SIMPLE WAYS TO BALANCE YOUR MIND, BODY, AND SOUL

When we think about health, diet and exercise are typically the first things that come to mind. However, good health isn't just about the physical body. Our mind and body are interconnected and affect each other tremendously.

For example, a stressful situation causing negative thoughts can lead to physical pain or illness. It's important to maintain a healthy balance between your mind, body, and soul by nurturing your whole self, including your physical, mental, emotional, and spiritual needs.

There are many things you can do in your daily life to achieve overall wellness. Here are 25 simple ways to begin cultivating a mind-body-soul balance.

1. Read and learn often. Your education shouldn't stop once you're out of school. Open your mind to new possibilities, beliefs, and interests by reading, taking online classes, watching documentaries, and attending workshops.

2. Meditate regularly. Meditation improves memory, attention, mood, immune system function, sleep, and creativity. All it takes is a few minutes a day to start reaping the benefits.

3. Practice yoga. Yoga is amazing for your overall health. It helps you build strength, coordination, and flexibility while calming your mind. It also encompasses the mind-body-soul connection.

4. Avoid sitting for extended periods of time. Try to stand or move around while you work, if possible. Too much sitting is linked to heart disease, diabetes, and a shortened lifespan.

5. Get at least 15 minutes of moderate to fast-paced exercise each day. Live close to work? Walk or ride your bike on nice days. Exercise is important for heart health, physical stamina, and mood.

6. Spend time outside. Now is the perfect time of year for hiking, boating, picnics, outdoor sports, foraging for wild foods, camping, and much more!

7. Add more plant-based foods to your diet. Eating lots of vegetables and fruit can help prevent chronic disease. Shop your local farmer's market for fresh, in-season produce.

8. Get involved in a volunteer organization or activism group. Use your voice or your talents to do some good in the world. We're all connected, and it's incredible to experience that connectedness when we work toward a common goal.

9. Fuel your passions. Set aside some time each day to do what makes your soul happy. Many of us work so much that we forget how great it feels to paint, dance, make music, write, garden, or swim.

10. Listen to music often. And sing along or dance!

11. Be grateful. Take some time each day to write or think about the things you're grateful for, like family, friends, pets, food, shelter, health, or the beauty of nature.

12. Be kind to everyone. This includes yourself!

13. Get enough sleep each night. And remember that you're never too old for naps.

14. Detoxify your beauty routine. Switch to natural products.

15. Get harsh chemical cleaners out of your house. Shop green cleaners, or make your own.

16. Find a career path that is meaningful to you. Chase your dreams, not riches.

17. Let go of the little things. If something won't matter tomorrow, don't let it ruin today.

18. Slow down. A little rest and relaxation when you're used to spending lots of time on the go can replenish your mind and body.

19. Stop people pleasing. There's a difference between being kind and being a doormat. If you spend too much time worrying about what others will think, you'll lose yourself and end up feeling miserable.

20. Cut major sources of stress out of your life. This includes unnecessary spending, clutter, a job you hate, or unhealthy relationships.

21. Avoid gossip and drama. Judging your neighbors and co-workers doesn't make you superior; it just makes you hard to trust.

22. Laugh often. If you take life to seriously, you're going to miss out on a whole lot of good times.

23. Travel and learn about other cultures. Do this as much as you can!

24. Forgive yourself for your past mistakes. Learn from the past, but don't let it destroy you.

25. Opt for natural remedies whenever you can. With the guidance of a holistic health practitioner, herbs, the right foods, and essential oils can be very healing and have fewer dangerous side effects than most pharmaceuticals.

INCONCLUSION

Whether they are for an exercise machine, a pharmaceutical product or a nutritional or herbal product, many health commercials have two elements in common: they offer "magic bullets," or quick fixes to health conditions, and the touted products address a purely physical level of being. I can't think of one conventional medical product whose advertising campaign offers a holistic or multi-dimensional approach to meeting health challenges. And, although complementary medicine is multi-dimensional by nature, the pills and potions are pushed in similarly one-dimensional ways. But deep, lasting changes in ingrained health patterns are rarely one-dimensional. And profound changes always entail movement on more than the physical level.

All life depends on a balance of elements or forces. Night and day. Oxygen and carbon dioxide. Activity and rest. Yin and yang. Where there is imbalance, systems operate out of synch and function is compromised. Human beings are not exempt from this e□uation. Think of the forces that support a human being in terms of the pillars of a triangle. For radiant health to occur in humans, a balance must exist on all three points of the triangle -- spirit, mind and body.

Body

Achieving and maintaining physical health is largely dependent on two lifestyle choices: nutrition and exercise. Except in cases where there is a functional or organic health limitation, appropriate food and exercise will control weight gain and maintain our physical systems in optimal condition.

Choice of exercise is a personal matter. The best exercise is one that raises the pulse rate above 120 beats per minute for more than 15 minutes, five days a week. Within this aerobic guideline, it really doesn't matter which exercise regimen you choose. Brisk walking will accomplish this goal, especially when carrying two to five pound weights in each hand so the upper body gets a workout while you are walking. Positive results will be achieved as long as you are consistent with an exercise pattern and avoid the obsessive behaviors that hurt, rather than help your body. Leave the "no pain, no gain," approach to testosterone-saturated locker rooms.

Nutrition is more difficult to get a hold on because of the misinformation and fad diets that flood the marketplace. Each person is biologically individuated, so eating according to a certain "type" really doesn't work for most people. There is no canned diet that will work for you as well as a diet that you develop based on feedback from your body and some common sense principles.

These principles include:

* Avoid fried foods.

* Eat red meat sparingly.

* Have at least 5 portions of fruit and vegetables a day.

* Lower your alcohol, sugar, salt and caffeine intake to as close to zero as you can.

* Discover which foods you are sensitive or allergic to and avoid them. The most common allergenic foods are dairy, wheat, corn, eggs and gluten-containing grains.

* Drink at least 8 glasses of pure water a day.

* Eat organically as much as you can and filter all bath, drinking and cooking water.

* Take as few supplements as you truly need.

* If you have difficulty in determining which diet works best for you, find a health practitioner who can assist you.

* Finally, when the body does need medical attention, look to non-toxic, holistic approaches before opting for pharmaceuticals.

Mind

The essential foundation of mind-body medicine is the recognition that for every experience in the mind, there is a corresponding change in the physiology and biochemistry of our body. We have a vast internal pharmacy that can be accessed through conscious choices we make in our lives. A key tenet of mind-body medicine is that health is not the mere absence of disease. Rather, it is the dynamic integration of our environment, body, mind and spirit.

Mind-body medicine regards as fundamental an approach that respects and enhances each person's capacity for self-knowledge and self-care and emphasizes techniques that are grounded in this approach.

These techniques include self-awareness, relaxation, meditation, mindfulness, exercise, diet, biofeedback, visual imagery, self-hypnosis and group support. It explores and integrates the healing practices of other cultures, such as acupuncture and acupressure, meditation and yoga, as well as alternative Western approaches including naturopathic medicine, herbalism, massage, musculo-skeletal manipulation, holistic repatterning energetic medicine and prayer. It views illness as an opportunity for personal growth and transformation and health care providers as catalysts and guides in this process.

Mind and body are not separate. They are in constant and dynamic interaction. The images, or mental programs," that reside in your mind dramatically influence your mood (emotions), your behaviors, and the physical state of your body. Because they exert a direct chemical effect on your brain, these images determine whether you feel tired or energetic, in vibrant health or in pain, creative or depressed, dynamic or anxious at any given time.

Spirit

Spirit is the most important of the levels of being, yet it is the most intangible. Spirit is the cosmic glue that holds all three levels together. It is the unifying force in nature. People who are secure in their spiritual lives have fewer fears and tend to deal with health challenges in more constructive ways.

Physicians who work with very ill people know two things about the role of spirit in challenging health conditions: the prognosis is much better and, when it inevitably comes, transition from the body is less fearful and traumatic when a person acknowledges that there is a power in the universe that is greater than themselves.

Incorporating Spirit as part of our daily experience is more than following some preordained set of rules, meditating for hours in lotus position or belonging to a church or religion. It means the recognition that there is a profound inner essence that doesn't pass when the body does. It also entails striving to live conscious lives in attunement with our highest vision, to the extent that we are able to. And it means a lifelong commitment to the conscious pursuit of growth and change.

Albert Einstein once said words to the effect that problems we face cannot always be solved on the same level on which they were created. To me, this means that only by developing new perspectives and growing in spirit can we truly weather the inner transformations that are required to cause shifts on the physical and mental/emotional levels.

For purposes of discussion in this article I have presented the three levels of being separately. In reality, the levels intertwine and blend into each other with no clear dividing lines. Holistic physicians always assess their patients in terms of "center of gravity." This means that we evaluate the presenting condition from both energetic and clinical perspectives to determine which level of being plays the strongest influence in the pattern of illness. We then taper our approach to the patient in an attempt to restore balance and assist in the processes of transformation and growth.

www.ingramcontent.com/pod-product-compliance
Lightning Source LLC
Chambersburg PA
CBHW060809260726
48660CB00002B/858